An Atlas of
STROKE

THE ENCYCLOPEDIA OF VISUAL MEDICINE SERIES

An Atlas of
STROKE

Peter F. Semple, MB, FRCP

Senior Lecturer and Consultant Physician
Department of Medicine & Therapeutics, Gardiner Institute
Western Infirmary, Glasgow, Scotland, UK

Foreword by

Justin A. Zivin, MD, PhD

Professor of Neurosciences, School of Medicine
University of California, San Diego
La Jolla, CA, USA

The Parthenon Publishing Group
International Publishers in Medicine, Science & Technology

NEW YORK   LONDON

Library of Congress Cataloging-in-Publication Data
Semple, Peter F.
     An atlas of stroke / Peter F. Semple : foreword by
Justin A. Zivin.
         p. cm. -- (The Encyclopedia of visual medicine series)
     Includes bibliographical references and index.
     ISBN 1-85070-738-3
     1. Cerebrovascular disease--Atlases. I. Title. II. Series.
     [DNLM: 1. Cerebrovascular Disorders--atlases. WL 17
     S473a 1997]
     RC388,5,S455 1997
     616.8'1--dc21
     DNLM/DLC
     for Library of Congress   97–25927
                                                           CIP
British Library Cataloguing in Publication Data
Semple, Peter F.
     An atlas of stroke. - (The Encyclopedia of visual
     medicine series)
     1. Cerebrovascular disease 2. Cerebrovascular disease -
     Diagnosis 3. Cerebrovascular disease - Treatment
     I. Title
     616.8'1
     ISBN 1-85070-738-3

Published in the USA by
The Parthenon Publishing Group Inc.
One Blue Hill Plaza
PO Box 1564, Pearl River
New York 10965, USA

Published in the UK and Europe by
The Parthenon Publishing Group Limited
Casterton Hall, Carnforth
Lancs. LA6 2LA, UK

Printed and bound in Spain by T.G. Hostench, S.A.

Contents

Foreword

Until about a quarter of a century ago, all that we physicians could do for the cerebrovascular patient was to classify the various types of strokes. The actual treatment of stroke was an unattainable dream. Diagnosis was occasionally extremely challenging, and localization was based on clinical rules that sometimes failed.

The first revolution in the management of patients with cerebrovascular disease came when imaging methods were markedly improved. There are now a number of techniques that are helpful, and even more sophisticated modalities can be anticipated in the future. Diagnosis is now rarely difficult to achieve and stroke localization is precise.

Around two decades ago, stroke therapy began to be truly effective. Until that time, many therapeutic decisions were based on anecdotal evidence and 'armchair speculation' of a type that has now been shown to be useless or even worse. More recently, laboratory investigations and well-conducted clinical trials have provided a scientific basis for stroke treatment. First to come from this knowledge were the various prophylactic therapies. Hypertension control was shown to be important.

This was followed by proof that antiplatelet therapy is useful. Subsequently, the roles of surgical therapies and anticoagulation have become more clearly defined. The most recent steps forward have been towards the development of effective acute stroke therapies.

Strokes are one of the most common causes of death and disability in many parts of the world, and there is increasing emphasis on the need for speed in initiation of therapy. Therefore, many types of physicians will need to become familiar and comfortable with dealing with this disease. With this atlas, Dr Semple has written a simple but up-to-date summary of the rapidly advancing field of clinical imaging technology for the diagnosis and management of stroke patients. This book should provide students and physicians who are not cerebrovascular specialists with a sound foundation for an understanding of modern diagnostic procedures and the current literature. The concept of stroke therapy is no longer an oxymoron, and dissemination of the information contained in this atlas should be helpful to those of us who care for such patients.

Justin A. Zivin
La Jolla

Acknowledgements

I am grateful to the following colleagues for generously allowing the use of their slides in this atlas:

Dr Fred Adams, Dr Michael Sproule, Dr Tom Barrie, Dr John Byrne, Professor Henry Dargie and Mr Ian Sim of the Western Infirmary, Glasgow, Scotland;

Dr Marie Callaghan of the Law Hospital, Carluke, Lanarkshire; and

Dr Donald Grossett and Dr Keith Muir of the Institute of Neurological Sciences, Southern General Hospital, Glasgow, Scotland.

I would also like to thank Dr Alan S. Cohen of the Boston University School of Medicine, Boston, Massachusetts, USA, who so kindly provided the histological slides of amyloid angiopathy.

Finally, I am grateful to my colleagues, medical illustrators and all the others who have helped to make the idea of this present volume a reality.

Preface

At the time I was training as a physician in the early seventies, the diagnosis of stroke was solely clinical, supplemented on occasions by lumbar punctures and angiography, both of which were often embarked upon with trepidation.

The advent of computed tomography in the early seventies changed everything, not least because the technology permitted rapid, accurate and immediate diagnosis of hemorrhage. In the eighties came magnetic resonance imaging, which has greatly extended the ability to diagnose ischemic stroke, and produces remarkable images of the living brain. At the same time, Doppler ultrasound has evolved into an indispensable technique for the diagnosis of carotid artery disease. Other non-invasive methods of imaging the vasculature of the brain are being improved by the day.

The routine care of the acute stroke patient has improved greatly since my early years as a practicing physician. Moreover, I believe that we are now on the threshold of an exciting new era when effective treatment will at last be possible, probably in the form of early thrombolysis and novel neuroprotective drugs. Such an era will be in sharp contrast to the atmosphere of nihilism that appeared to prevail during earlier years.

The prevention of stroke by the use of antihypertensive and antithrombotic agents is now firmly established, and supported by incontrovertible evidence of efficacy. The main challenge remaining is to ensure that appropriate and effective pharmaceutical treatment is delivered to those at particular risk due to high blood pressure and atrial fibrillation, among other medical conditions.

The images of stroke now available from modern investigative technologies are striking and lend themselves particularly well to visual display in an atlas. *An Atlas of Stroke* is a logical extension from my earlier book, *An Atlas of Hypertension*.

I hope that this present atlas, as with its earlier 'partner', will prove to be a useful aid to those clinicians who are involved in the management of patients with vascular disorders.

Peter F. Semple
Glasgow

Section 1 A Review of Stroke

Epidemiology

Louis Pasteur sustained a left hemiparesis due to stroke at the age of 43 years. Fortunately, his intellect was apparently not impaired as he continued his celebrated research on microorganisms which culminated in the famous description of immunization against rabies.

Stroke, or apoplexy as it was once known, is the third leading cause of death in the developed world. It is, however, perhaps better known as a major cause of disability, accounting for no less than 5% of all monetary expenditure on health.

The condition is usually relatively easy to recognize clinically, as reflected by the definition of the World Health Organization: '...rapidly developing clinical signs of focal (or global) disturbance of cerebral function with symptoms lasting 24 hours or longer or leading to death with no apparent cause other than of vascular origin.' This definition encompasses subarachnoid hemorrhage, a distinctive condition with a unique pathophysiology and treatment.

Based on surveys of incidence and survival in the United Kingdom, the prevalence of stroke in the general population is 500–700 / 100 000 population, of whom at least half are left physically disabled or intellectually impaired[1]. The incidence increases exponentially with age from around 200 / 100 000 in the decade spanning the age of 60 years to around 3000 / 100 000 after age 85 years. There is some variation from country to country so that, after age 65 years, almost 90% of deaths are caused by stroke[2,3].

In most developed countries, the rate of mortality has fallen progressively over the century, with Japan showing a particularly steep decline. The annual rate of fall in the United States has tended to be around 5% in recent years, which appears to be due more to a reduction in case–fatality rate rather than in incidence. The current 1-year case–fatality rate is approximately 42%. Small cohort studies suggest that the incidence fell in eastern parts of the USA between the late 1940s and 1970s, and a similar decline was observed in Japan over the decade spanning the 1960s. In contrast, there is evidence from Eastern Europe to suggest that the incidence in those aged <70 years may in fact be increasing, despite the expected reduction in case–fatality rate[4].

Apparent increases in incidence in the USA more recently[5] must be viewed with some skepticism as diagnosis has improved with the advent of computed tomography (CT), and with the advances in this and other imaging techniques. Secular trends are always subject to potential bias due to changes in clinical practice and more subtle changes in diagnostic criteria. Furthermore, any changes in incidence and case–fatality rate must be viewed in the light of demographic changes resulting from increases in life expectancy.

It has been estimated that the increase of patients experiencing first stroke will be around 30% over the next few decades until the year 2020[1]. The WHO-sponsored MONICA project has established stroke registration in representative groups of the populations of 15 countries since 1984. The information is linked to the collection of data on risk factors and other cardiovascular events, and should provide a better idea of the more recent trends in incidence. In general and across different countries, it appears that stroke mortality tends to be higher where coronary heart disease mortality is lower.

The burden on the community is heavy. In particular, the costs of managing acute stroke are likely to increase now that there is good evidence to suggest that acute stroke units linked to a wider range of imaging techniques can reduce case–fatality rates. Around one-fifth of the patients who survive stroke require institutional care for the remainder of their lives. Stroke is also the terminal event for many elderly patients who are already disabled or in care so that up to 40% of stroke patients die in hospital.

Classification

Intracranial hemorrhage is easily detected on CT, but is a relatively infrequent cause of stroke; at present, bleeding accounts for around 10% of admissions to an acute stroke unit both in Europe and in North America. The pattern in the Far East is somewhat different, with intracerebral hemorrhage accounting for around 25% of strokes in Japan. Such differences are probably the result of different patterns of risk factors in the respective populations, particularly arterial blood pressure, and plasma levels of cholesterol and other lipid fractions.

A reliable subclassification of cerebral infarction is more difficult to determine because various processes lead to interruption of blood flow, including atherosclerosis and thrombosis, small-vessel disease and embolism, which itself can be further divided into cardiac embolism and artery-to-artery embolism.

Various schemes for a clinical classification of stroke have been devised, supplemented or confirmed by information from CT, magnetic resonance imaging (MRI), carotid duplex Doppler ultrasonography or other imaging techniques.

The Oxford scheme of clinical classification (see Section 2, Figure 1) is widely used[6], and divides infarcts into carotid or anterior circulation infarcts (ACI) and vertebrobasilar or posterior circulation infarcts (POCI). The ACI are further subdivided into lesions which affect both cortical and subcortical structures, resulting in hemiplegia, hemisensory loss, hemianopia and higher cortical dysfunction, and are referred to as total ACI or TACI. Events which cause only partial cortical deficits, such as aphasia, are referred to as partial ACI or PACI.

The Oxford classification is useful in terms of prognosis as total syndromes have a poor prognosis for survival and functional outcome. However, the scheme does not distinguish between embolic and atherothrombotic events.

Since the pioneering studies of C. Miller Fisher in Boston, lacunar infarcts (or LACI in the Oxford system) have been delineated by clinical criteria based on neuroanatomical principles[7]. Lacunar infarcts were originally defined as events resulting from occlusion of single perforating end arteries 50–200 Å in diameter. The definition remains useful in clinical practice in terms of prognosis and definition of subgroups for clinical trials. Its main weakness is the incomplete relationship to pathophysiology as small deep infarcts may also be a result of atherosclerosis as well as of the characteristic small-vessel disease of hypertension and diabetes mellitus. Some posterior circulation infarcts are lacunar and share a common pathophysiology.

Other classification schemes have been devised and are based more on pathological, rather than neuroanatomical, mechanisms. These include that derived from data emerging from the Stroke Data Bank Study[8] and that of the National Institute of Neurological Disorders and Stroke[9] (see Section 2, Figures 1 and 2). Both systems infer causality on the basis of the presence of potential cardiac sources of embolism and of proximal arterial stenoses. In clinical practice, however, such a distinction is not easily achieved and there is often no entirely reliable method of verification.

Investigation

Transient ischemic attacks

The time-honored definition of a transient ischemic attack (TIA) is an episode of focal loss of cerebral function or vision lasting < 24 h due to a temporary interruption of blood supply. A TIA is a presentiment of stroke as around one in three patients who present with TIA will develop completed stroke within 3 years. The clinical syndrome identifies a group of patients in some of whom stroke may be prevented by treatment of a carotid stenosis or by institution of antithrombotic measures or, less frequently, by diagnosis of conditions such as systemic lupus erythematosus or necrotizing arteritis.

Symptoms of cerebral dysfunction that are not focal, such as confusion, loss of consciousness or loss of vision associated with a reduced level of consciousness, are not considered TIAs. Likewise, isolated symptoms that may have other causes, such as vertigo and disturbances of balance, dysarthria and dysphagia, scintillating scotomas and sensory symptoms confined to part of a limb or the face, are also not classified under the rubric.

Migraine and seizures are often considered in the differential diagnosis, although migraine with aura may present particular difficulties. In migraine, there tends to be a slow progression of symptoms from part to part over a period of up to 30 min, and affected patients tend to be relatively young. Headache is not a particularly useful discriminant. In contrast, focal seizures tend to cause 'positive' rather than 'negative' symptoms, and have a characteristic rapid progression from a distal point in the limb or face to become more widespread.

A TIA due to a critical carotid stenosis may occasionally cause shaking or tremor of a limb which may be mistaken for a focal seizure. TIAs in the carotid territory tend to cause visual loss in one eye, aphasia or unilateral motor and / or sensory symptoms. However, some posterior circulation events may have similar presentations.

Sensory or motor symptoms that are bilateral suggest that ischemia in the vertebrobasilar territory is highly likely as do blindness, diplopia, vertigo and loss of balance.

Patient history and clinical examination may give useful pointers as to the mechanism of TIAs. Bruits may be detected over the carotid artery and, less commonly, the subclavian artery, but tend not to be either sensitive or specific. Systolic murmurs transmitted from the aortic valve may lead to false-positive results.

The familiar description of symptoms of hemispheric ischemia or amaurosis fugax should prompt carotid Doppler ultrasonography. In such cases, CT and MRI are of limited value for investigation as it is often difficult to date stroke events with certainty, and brain-stem infarcts are difficult to visualize with CT. Although these imaging modalities are a necessary component of patient investigation, most clinicians continue to define the condition solely on the basis of clinical criteria.

Atrial fibrillation, cardiac murmurs or evidence of myocardial infarction should raise suspicions of cardiogenic embolism, and electrocardiography (ECG) and echocardiography may provide similar clues.

Transthoracic echocardiography is especially effective in identifying left ventricular dysfunction and ventricular sources of embolism, but has limited value in detecting thrombus in the atria and atrial appendages, for which the transesophageal (TOE) approach provides much better definition. TOE is also able to render good definition of the aorta and may give a diagnosis of dissection or reveal evidence of a protruding atheroma, a potential source of atheroembolism.

Artery-to-artery embolism may give rise to refractile deposits in the retinal arterioles, so-called Hollenhorst plaques, which tend to be visualized at points of arteriolar bifurcation. Finally, uncontrolled hypertension may be a pointer to an incipient lacunar event.

Brain imaging using CT or MRI may reveal evidence of previous events. MRI is better than CT in detecting brain-stem infarction and small deep hemispheric infarcts. Cerebrovascular ischemic changes can be detected earlier with MRI, although small bright signals may be present and give false-positive results. The requirement for the patient to remain still and recumbent in an MRI scanner is a major limitation on acute use, and claustrophobia may sometimes cause difficulties.

The presence of infarcts between areas supplied by different cerebral arteries may be an indication of a period of reduced cerebral perfusion or suggest the presence of a proximal arterial stenosis. The most easily recognizable border-zone or 'watershed' infarcts are located between the territories of the middle and anterior, and middle and posterior, cerebral arteries, although variability in blood supply from one individual to another can lead to difficulties in recognition. Infarcts at the junctions of deep and superficial middle cerebral arterial branches, and in the cerebellar hemisphere, are more difficult to recognize.

Ultrasound is widely used as a screening test for carotid atherosclerosis and stenosis, and is particularly appropriate in the investigation of TIAs of the anterior cerebral circulation and eye[10,11]. Nowadays, carotid revascularization may not require prior contrast arteriography[12] and non-invasive approaches such as MRI angiography and spiral CT may be useful in defining arterial anatomy.

Over the last 20 years, there has been a major increase in the technology of carotid ultrasonography. Advances have included increased selectivity and sensitivity of pulsed Doppler ultrasound, the addition of color imaging and improved resolution.

Duplex sonography describes the combination of ultrasound imaging of the vessel wall with pulse-gated Doppler. The procedures are linked so that the two-dimensional real-time image can be used to locate the area of interest for the Doppler part of the study. The duplex system allows the operator to switch easily from one mode to the other. Doppler signatures are digitized and visually displayed.

Occlusion of the internal carotid artery can now be diagnosed with added confidence by Doppler with color-coded flow velocities (CDI). Additional information regarding plaque morphology, and especially ulceration and hemorrhage, can be obtained with an acceptable degree of accuracy. The technique has also been used to quantify intima–media thickness (IMT) as an index of atherosclerosis in clinical trials. However, a major limitation of all ultrasound systems is the inability to detect 'tandem' lesions in the carotid siphon or middle cerebral artery. MRI angiography may be a useful non-invasive method for detecting middle cerebral artery stenosis. With Doppler, there is a small risk (1–10%) that high-grade internal carotid stenoses may be mistaken for total occlusion and, thus, many prefer to make a precise assessment of arterial anatomy with contrast angiography.

The mechanism of TIAs in carotid stenosis is thought to involve artery-to-artery embolism in the majority of cases, although ischemic events secondary to hemodynamic changes are seen. The latter tend to be stereotyped and are liable to be provoked by reductions in arterial pressure or cardiac output.

The major clinical trials of carotid endarterectomy for symptomatic internal carotid stenosis that have guided current clinical practice are the European Carotid Stenosis Trial (ECST), and the CASANOVA and NASCET trials from North America published in 1991[13–15]. More recently, the Asymptomatic Carotid Atherosclerosis Study (ACAS) on the surgical management of asymptomatic stenosis has reported positive results[16].

There is a general consensus that surgical treatment can provide benefit in suitable patients who have severe symptomatic stenosis (>70%), but there is much less agreement regarding the cost-effectiveness of treating asymptomatic patients. For a single ischemic event and compared with medical treatment, surgery reduces the risk of ipsilateral stroke at 2 years from 19% to 9%, and that of recurrent events from 41% to 11%[17].

Patients with symptomatic coronary artery disease and symptomatic or asymptomatic carotid disease present a particular management dilemma. Current evidence is incomplete, but carotid surgery followed by coronary surgery or a combined operation appear to minimize the risk of stroke whereas the two-stage procedure increases the risk of myocardial infarction and death.

In addition, there are a number of methodological problems because of the different systems used to quantify the degree of arterial stenosis in the different trials. All of the various methods used calculated the percentage of minimal residual lumen (MRL), but different denominators were applied, such as the distal lumen (DL) diameter or 'normal' bulb diameter. Further uncertainty has resulted from the use of various definitions for the carotid bulb and sinus, and it has also been suggested that the diameter of the proximal common carotid artery may be a better reference point.

In practice, most clinicians use the diameter of the MRL divided by the diameter of the DL, where the walls are parallel. However, diameter stenosis in one plane is not linearly related to a cross-sectional area. Therefore, a 50% diameter stenosis approximates to a 75% area stenosis. The relationship between angiographic and Doppler measurements in a given laboratory is not always well-defined and may be another potential pitfall in the assessment of severity.

Distal stenosis and restenosis after surgery may be treated by angioplasty and stent, but the roles of these newer techniques are currently still not fully defined. A prospective randomized clinical trial comparing surgery with angioplasty and stent insertion is necessary before the uses of these less invasive techniques can be assessed. Uncontrolled use of catheter-based methods may not be appropriate at present.

Earlier hopes that intravenous digital subtraction angiography might replace intra-arterial contrast injection have not been realized because the quality of the former image tends to be less than optimal, especially if left ventricular function is impaired. MRI angiography and spiral CT are promising, but large-scale experience has not yet been accumulated and image definition remains inferior to that achieved with intra-arterial contrast injection.

Another non-invasive screening technique for internal carotid stenosis is ocular pneumoplethysmography, although the method has not found much favor. It is recognized that surgeons who carry out endarterectomy need to perform sufficient numbers of procedures to verify the rate of complications in terms of operative morbidity; stroke morbidity should be around 2% and certainly less than 5%.

The most important approach to the medical management of carotid stenosis is the use of antiplatelet drugs and aspirin in particular. In the most recent meta-analysis of stroke risk reduction in patients with TIAs or minor ischemic stroke, antiplatelet drugs resulted in a 2% absolute-risk reduction and a 23% odds reduction in terms of non-fatal stroke[18]. Furthermore, the new antiplatelet drug clopidogrel may be more effective than aspirin[19]. The optimal

dose of aspirin for stroke prophylaxis remains the subject of intense debate[20,21].

Other experimental techniques may provide useful information regarding cerebral perfusion distal to an extracranial or intracranial arterial stenosis. Changes in flow velocity within the middle cerebral artery, as determined by transcranial Doppler ultrasound, may allow assessment of hemispheric perfusion reserve. The reserve will be reduced if flow velocity remains unaffected by elevation of arterial carbon dioxide partial pressure (pCO_2), which is accomplished simply by breath-holding.

Another technique for quantifying hemispheric blood flow is single-photon emission computed tomography (SPECT), which uses the gamma-emitting properties of radioligands such as technetium 99m (^{99m}Tc)-hexamethylpropylene amine oxide (HMPAO) or ^{123}I (radioiodine)-amphetamine, and produces images using a standard gamma camera. Scanning during ischemia may provide information concerning distribution. Investigation can be carried out before and after manipulation of pCO_2 by acetazolamide treatment to allow estimation of perfusion reserve. These techniques are not as yet used routinely in the investigation of TIAs.

The ischemic penumbra

Deficient blood supply to a part of the brain causes reduced function of neurons and glia which may progress to cell death and permanent dysfunction. The biochemical mechanisms of ischemia and cell death have been extensively investigated, focusing on strategies and treatments that may prevent or attenuate permanent damage. Brain ischemia affects not only neurotransmitters, receptors, membrane ion channels and processes of phosphorylation, but may also have an effect on the generation of toxic free radicals as well as on modification of gene expression and regulation. Neurons and glial cells are affected in different ways, and there is particular interest in processes that may be reversible.

Certain neurons, namely, the pyramidal neurons in the CA1 and CA4 zones of the hippocampus, and some of the neurons in the caudate nucleus, are most vulnerable to ischemic death. Histopathology after cardiac arrest in animals has provided information regarding the vulnerability of neurons to global ischemia, and focal ischemia could be expected to have similar effects. A period of 60 min or less of focal ischemia is sufficient to cause infarction and necrosis of neurons and glia, but there is a surrounding zone of spared glia. Around the central area of necrosis is an area of ischemia causing cell dysfunction of variable degrees, some of which are potentially reversible. Severe ischemia causes persistent depolarization of neurons, but there is a surrounding zone of only intermittent depolarization. This area is often described as the ischemic penumbra and may vary considerably in size.

Severe ischemia causes depletion of adenosine triphosphate (ATP), but energy failure is probably not the immediate cause of cell necrosis. Other downstream factors may kill cells either immediately or after a period of time, even when the initial ATP levels have been restored. Generation of toxic free radical species as a result of ischemia and reperfusion may be a critical mechanism determining cell injury and death, but acidosis due in part to lactate accumulation is also a mediator of cell injury, particularly in the neuroglia.

Failure of energy supplies to the ion pumps that maintain membrane potential levels results in a collapse of gradients of sodium, potassium and calcium across cells, and an increase in intracellular calcium, with resultant calcium mediator-enzyme activation; this has also been implicated as a cause of cell death. Thus far, however, it has been disappointing that attempts to prevent cell death by blockade of calcium entry or intracellular release of calcium have not been entirely successful.

Intracellular and excitatory amino acids such as glutamate and aspartate are released in response to ischemia. Various studies have provided evidence that calcium entry through glutamate-regulated membrane channels is detrimental to survival. Several receptors appear to be involved, including the quisqualate and NMDA (N-methyl-D-aspartate) receptor complexes which are linked to calcium entry channels.

In animal models of acute ischemic stroke, ultimate infarct size can be substantially attenuated by the administration of several experimental agents either before or after arterial occlusion. In addition, as in the heart, there appears to be an ischemic tolerance phenomenon[22]. Tolerance of ischemia in the brain apparently develops more slowly and persists for longer than in the heart, and probably requires the synthesis of new protein.

A major challenge for clinical trials is to administer potentially effective agents as early as possible after the onset of ischemia and to deliver the drug in adequate concentrations to the tissue that has a reduced blood supply. For clinical trials of neuro-protective drugs, the inhomogeneous nature of acute stroke in humans creates further difficulties. Ischemic stroke may be the result of large-artery thrombosis, small-vessel disease affecting subcortical white matter, embolism from the heart or proximal arteries and various other rare vascular events, including arterial dissection and arteritis.

Cardioembolism

Embolism from the heart as a cause of stroke was first recognized nearly 150 years ago. The entity has attracted increasing attention during the last decade because of several clinical trials which have clearly demonstrated the benefit of anticoagulant treatment in preventing stroke in patients with potential cardiac sources, especially atrial fibrillation.

At present, there is no certain method for differentiating embolic stroke from other types of arterial occlusion. It has been estimated that embolism accounts for 15–20% of clinical stroke events[23,24]. Mode of onset is sometimes helpful in that slow or stuttering onset is clearly not consistent with an embolic etiology. Major risk factors include atrial fibrillation, anterior myocardial infarction, a poorly contracting left ventricle[25] and mitral valve disease.

The advent of TOE has given impetus to the search for potential sources in the heart. In series of patients with acute stroke, potential embolic sources have been recognized in up to one-third of patients[26]. Unfortunately, patients with a risk of embolism due to atrial fibrillation often have concomitant ischemic or hypertensive heart disease and cranial or extracranial atherosclerosis.

Embolism tends to be more frequently a cause of stroke in the very young, who should be subjected to careful cardiac investigation. However, embolism is also relatively frequent in elderly patients with stroke, a group in whom the recognition of embolism is much more difficult and where the risks of anticoagulant treatment must be carefully weighed against the known benefits.

The type and location of infarction, as seen on CT, is sometimes helpful in diagnosis. Embolism from the atria or ventricles tends to cause cortical infarcts, including some of the middle cerebral artery branch syndromes, especially occlusion at the first branch of the lower division, resulting in Wernicke's aphasia, as well as posterior cerebral artery occlusion. Striatocapsular infarcts are also likely to have an embolic cause as sudden occlusion of the cerebral artery stem will block the orifices of the lenticulo-striate arteries with relative sparing of superficial middle cerebral artery territories.

Smaller subcortical events of lacunar type are not currently believed to result from embolism. The distribution of injected microspheres in experimental animals offers some support to this view.

Early hemorrhagic transformation of cerebral infarcts is somewhat more likely after embolic stroke, although reperfusion and hemorrhage may also develop in large infarcts caused by atherosclerosis. Indeed, nearly 40% of middle cerebral artery infarcts show some evidence of reperfusion at 48 h.

Multiple cortical infarcts in an elderly patient in the presence of a cardiac source strongly suggest an embolic cause whereas embolism from heart valves tends to cause TIAs or amaurosis fugax. In patients with mechanical prosthetic heart valves, prophylaxis may be best if warfarin is combined with low-dose aspirin. The benefits of such a combination appear to outweigh the increased risk of gastrointestinal bleeding[27], although some argue that optimal control of anticoagulation with warfarin alone achieves the same results.

The risk of embolism in young patients is probably increased in the presence of mitral valve prolapse, patent foramen ovale and atrial septal aneurysm[28]. Transcranial Doppler sonography after intravenous injection of microbubbles, perhaps supplemented by cough or the Valsalva maneuver, is useful for detecting those who have patent foramen ovale or, alternatively, TOE[29].

Other conditions associated with an increased risk of embolic stroke include marantic endocarditis, Libman–Sacks endocarditis due to systemic lupus erythematosus with antiphospholipid antibodies and calcification of the mitral annulus. Patients who have aortic plaques > 4 mm in thickness at TOE have a high risk of stroke, and some of these events may be embolic[30].

The results of several major randomized trials of anticoagulation in primary and secondary prevention of stroke in patients with non-rheumatic atrial fibrillation have been reported during the last decade and have transformed clinical practice[31–36]. Without anticoagulant treatment, 5–8% of patients > 60 years of age with atrial fibrillation showed evidence of an ischemic brain event every year.

Warfarin anticoagulation to achieve an international normalized ratio of between 1.5 and 4.0 reduces the risk by around 20% with less than 2.5% of significant bleeding events per year. Aspirin is apparently somewhat less effective, but still confers benefit compared with no treatment. It is still important to recognize that indiscriminate use of warfarin in elderly patients with atrial fibrillation may cause bleeding complications. For this reason, some of the trials used rigorous exclusion criteria so that only a relatively small proportion of patients with atrial fibrillation were admitted.

Younger patients with lone atrial fibrillation appear to have a low risk of stroke. Not surprisingly, previous stroke or TIA, fibrillation, recent heart failure or a history of hypertension defines groups with a relatively high risk of embolic events.

The optimal level of anticoagulation for secondary prevention in non-rheumatic atrial fibrillation appears to be at an international normalized ratio of 3.0[37]. All patients > 60 years of age should receive antithrombotic treatment unless there is a definite contraindication.

In the first 2 weeks following myocardial infarction, 1–5% of patients have an ischemic stroke. The risk is particularly high after anterior events and if there are areas of dyskinesia[38]. Full anticoagulation with heparin prevents ischemic events after anterior infarction, and aspirin treatment reduces the incidence. The combination of low-dose heparin with aspirin appears to reduce the risk of ischemic stroke to 1% or less shortly after infarction, although full-dose heparin treatment is generally preferred.

Thrombolytic treatment alone apparently does not have much effect on the frequency of ischemic stroke caused by mural thrombus. An appreciable risk of embolism (around 10% per year) is found in patients with continuing evidence of ventricular thrombus. In these patients, low-intensity anticoagulation with warfarin is the best treatment.

An important unresolved difficulty in the treatment of patients with cardiogenic embolic stroke is the optimal timing and nature of anticoagulant therapy. The risk of hemorrhagic transformation of large cerebral infarcts is high, and will most likely become visible on CT between 12 h and 4 days after onset.

Anticoagulation increases the risk of late hemorrhage, which may result in deterioration of neurological status. The current practice is to defer anticoagulant treatment for a variable period of up to 10 days in high-risk patients with large infarcts, but there is an urgent need for clinical trials to inform practice. Any risk of immediate hemorrhagic transformation has to be balanced against the risk of further embolism, which appears to be approximately 10% over 2 weeks, although there is wide variation across series.

Mode of onset is sometimes helpful in determining other causes of ischemic stroke. The classical stuttering onset occurs in a small proportion of atherothrombotic events and, in some cases, lacunar strokes may show a slow progressive worsening of symptoms over 24–48 h.

Headache after cerebral infarction may indicate embolism, but the degree of discrimination is low as up to 30% of patients with ischemic stroke have headache. The peak incidence of ischemic stroke, as with hemorrhage, is between 0800 h and 1000 h, a period when arterial pressures tend to be high. A potential confounding factor in these analyses is the inclusion of individuals whose onset of stroke is some time before awakening.

Unfortunately, CT is of limited value in the diagnosis of early ischemic stroke, and changes are often undetectable or subtle in the early hours. Full delineation of the area of infarction is best after 7–10 days. The newer-generation scanners are better able to detect the early changes of infarction, such as effacement of the distinction between white and gray matter, and blurring of the normal sulcal patterns. Periods of isodensity occurring around 3

days after infarction occasionally cause difficulties. Infarcts in the brain stem tend to be poorly visualized, but those in the cerebellar hemispheres are reasonably well-defined.

MRI, and T_2-weighted scans in particular, are better able to localize brain-stem ischemic events and small deep infarcts or lacunar infarcts. Contrast enhancement with gadolinium increases sensitivity, but may give false-positive results.

Ischemic changes can be seen on T_2-weighted MRI early in the development of ischemic stroke but, at this stage, MRI is less reliable in differentiating hemorrhage from infarction. The suggestion that SPECT may be a better predictor of outcome than clinical scoring has yet to be confirmed.

The extent of cerebral infarction after atherothrombotic occlusion varies widely among subjects even when the same artery has been occluded. Internal carotid artery occlusion may cause devastating hemispheric infarction in some patients, but only a TIA, or no symptoms at all, in others.

The extent of infarction after carotid or middle cerebral artery occlusion clearly depends on the adequacy of the collaterals. The size of the posterior communicating artery on the relevant side has been identified as an important determinant of the extent of infarction. The collateral circulation established during a preexisting period of arterial stenosis may also be important.

In contrast to findings in white Europeans, occlusion of the middle cerebral artery stem is a relatively common cause of atherosclerotic stroke in Eastern Asia and Africa. The result is widespread subcortical infarction in the territories of the lenticulostriate and other perforating arteries, with or without major infarction of the superficial middle cerebral artery territory.

In rats with experimentally induced middle cerebral artery occlusion, the extent of infarction is apparently much greater in animals with certain genetic strains of hypertension, but the determinants of this susceptibility have not yet been ascertained. It is fairly certain that structural changes in cerebral arteries as a result of hypertension limit collateral blood flow after vascular occlusion.

The stress of major stroke often increases plasma concentrations of glucose, and high plasma glucose levels appear to have an adverse effect on infarct size and prognosis. Blood pressures are commonly raised immediately post-stroke, with loss of the usual nocturnal dip. However, the safety of anti-hypertensive therapy during this phase, when autoregulatory mechanisms are improved, is not established.

Care in an acute stroke unit compared with a general medical ward has been shown to reduce mortality and improve functional outcome[39–42]. The individual components of care have not been identified, but maintenance of an airway, proper assessment of swallowing, and better management of fluid and glucose metabolism are likely to be involved. It is estimated that the minimum increase in staff in a general ward compared with a dedicated stroke unit is 1.0 for the number of nurses, and 0.3 each for physiotherapists and occupational therapists, for every six patients.

Lacunar strokes

Small infarcts deep in the cerebral hemispheres and in the brain stem caused by occlusion of perforating end arteries originating in the circle of Willis, and of the proximal middle, posterior cerebral and basilar arteries, are often described as 'lacunar'. The term derives from gross pathology where a lacune refers to a small slit-like space usually in the basal ganglia or basis pontis. The typical appearance of lacunar strokes may be the result of areas of infarction that are 2–15 mm in diameter, but resorption of small areas of hemorrhage may produce an identical appearance. Lacunes may develop silently in many instances.

A number of well-defined stroke syndromes – termed lacunar syndromes – are believed to result from occlusion of a single penetrating artery causing infarcts that are 0.5–2 cm in diameter. Approximately 10–20% of strokes in Europe and in the USA are lacunar syndromes.

Historically, this type of stroke was linked causally to hypertensive small-vessel disease, although some doubt has been cast on this simple concept. The syndrome may be caused by atherosclerosis. C. Miller Fisher originally described a type of medial degeneration in affected vessels which he termed 'lipohyalinosis', but the pathological process leading to most of the small-vessel occlusion remains under dispute. Furthermore, the relationship to the more familiar larger-artery atherosclerosis remains poorly defined.

The most commonly encountered lacunar syndrome is pure motor hemiplegia, affecting the face, arm and leg, as a result of infarction in the internal capsule or in the basis pontis. In some cases, infarction is situated in the corona radiata, cerebral peduncle or, less commonly, medulla oblongata. A relatively high proportion of these small deep infarcts are not visualized on CT, which creates further difficulties in making accurate neuro-anatomical correlations. MRI has greater sensitivity, but may produce a high proportion of false-positive results, and may not allow differentiation between infarction and areas of demyelination caused by other processes.

The clinical definition of the lacunar syndromes is dependent on the proximity of motor fibers to the face, arm and leg within the relevant areas of white matter and especially the posterior internal capsule. A proportion of patients with partial syndromes, and especially with weakness confined to the arm and leg, have small deep infarcts. However, expanding the definition to include patients with brachiofacial weakness will significantly increase the proportion of patients in whom cortical infarcts are found.

By definition, aphasia, visuospatial neglect, agnosia, apraxia and visual-field deficits do not occur in lacunar syndromes, but may be present as a result of larger striatocapsular infarcts, which probably have a different etiology. In comparison to hemiplegia caused by cortical infarcts, pure motor hemiplegia due to small deep infarcts carries a considerably better prognosis in terms of recovery of functional capacity.

Pure sensory stroke is another lacunar syndrome that accounts for <10% of all clinical lacunar syndromes. They are caused by very small infarcts in the thalamus, the bulk of which is supplied by branches of the posterior cerebral artery, except for the anterior pole. Clinically, patients often present with symptoms of widespread unilateral paresthesia and, on occasions, there is an element of dissociated sensory loss. Pure sensory stroke may evolve after several months into a distressing syndrome of chronic pain in the affected side.

The original concept of lacunar infarction did not include sensorimotor stroke because of the separate blood supplies to the thalamus and posterior internal capsule. However, it is now clear that such strokes can be caused by small deep infarcts. Diagnostic precision in terms of locating sensorimotor strokes is not as accurate as with either pure motor or pure sensory strokes.

Other classical lacunar syndromes are homolateral ataxia, and crural paresis and dysarthria with clumsy hand, both of which may be encompassed in the term 'ataxic hemiparesis' and may be caused by small infarcts in the basis pontis. The syndrome is not common, and dysmetria may be difficult to detect clinically in a weak limb. Some small brainstem infarcts with a central location may be caused by small-vessel disease, but clinical definition is difficult. Warning TIAs quite often occur before the definitive event in lacunar stroke.

Clinical distinction of lacunar infarcts from small deep hemorrhages is rarely possible without CT. As hypertensive cerebral hemorrhage and lacunar infarction both originate in small deep perforators, a common etiological mechanism is likely. Because lacunar infarcts are small, deep and distant from pain-sensitive tissues, headache is unusual.

Intracerebral hemorrhage

Bleeding into the brain as a cause of acute stroke was described in as early as the sixteenth and seventeenth centuries, but the burgeoning pathological description in the nineteenth century firmly defined hemorrhage as a cause of stroke. Charcot and Duret dubbed the lateral lenticulostriate artery the 'artery of cerebral hemorrhage'. Bouchard and Charcot recognized the origin of bleeding from microaneurysms as early as 1868 at virtually the same time that Mohamed at Guy's Hospital in London began to recognize clinical hypertension.

A completely reliable distinction of hemorrhage from infarction in patients was not possible until the development of CT in the early 1970s. In the acute situation, CT is unrivalled as a method of diagnosis although MRI, which is able to detect hemosiderin, is more useful than CT in the chronic stage. Contrast angiography is only necessary to define aneurysms and vascular malformation.

Hematomas commonly increase in size in the hour or two after admission and may continue to increase for 12 h or longer. Deeply placed hematomas, especially in the putamen, are characteristic of hypertension. Not surprisingly, most episodes of bleeding start at times of the day when arterial pressures are high. This is also the case with subarachnoid hemorrhage due to aneurysm rupture.

In recent years, a novel pathology has been shown to cause more superficial or lobar cerebral hemorrhages, events which may account for more than 50% of bleeds in Europe and North America, and a high proportion of events in the elderly. Many are now known to be caused by rupture of vessels with amyloid deposits in the walls[43]. Amyloid shows a predilection for the cortical veins, arteries and vessels of the leptomeninges. Hemorrhage caused by amyloid angiopathy is increasingly common in patients aged 60 years and over. Bleeding is often initiated at the junction of gray and white matter.

Amyloid deposition tends to spare vessels supplying the basal ganglia and brain stem, although it may be present in the vessels of the cerebellar hemispheres. Bleeding is sometimes multicentric and, in some instances, premonitory symptoms resembling TIAs have been described. These symptoms may be due to areas of ischemia and infarction, or to minute areas of hemorrhage triggering waves of spreading depression, as in migraine. When amyloid angiopathy is the cause of cerebral hemorrhage, recurrence is likely.

Other causes of lobar hemorrhage include vascular malformations and some metastatic cerebral tumors, malignant melanoma in particular, and abuse of sympathomimetic drugs such as cocaine.

Overtreatment with anticoagulants may present similarly, and there is some evidence that bleeding after thrombolytic treatment of myocardial infarction may be predominantly lobar. The safety of thrombolytic therapy for acute stroke with symptoms for >3 h has not been established. The average risk of intracerebral hemorrhage in treated patients is around 10%, or three-and-one-half times that of controls[44].

The clinical symptoms of lobar hemorrhage, but not deep hemorrhage, are headache and early seizure accompanied by few signs of chronic hypertension. Vomiting is a powerful predictor of hemorrhage in supratentorial stroke; it occurs especially in cases of hemorrhage into the caudate nucleus. Proximity of the caudate nucleus to the ventricular system predisposes to rupture into the lateral ventricles, which leads to an abrupt increase in intracranial pressure. Blood pressures after intracerebral hemorrhage tend to be higher than after cerebral infarction.

Hypertensive cerebral hemorrhage most often originates in the putamen. The classical findings in large putaminal hemorrhages are hemiplegia, hemisensory loss, hemianopia, conjugate deviation of the eyes towards the side of the lesion, impaired consciousness, aphasia or contralateral neglect depending on hemispheric dominance. Hyperreflexia may be present at an early stage. Smaller anterior and posterior lesions tend to have a better prognosis than those located more centrally, but coma carries a very poor prognosis.

Thalamic hemorrhage with pressure on the midbrain tends to cause abnormalities of vertical gaze wherein the eyes are deviated downwards and inwards. Sensory deficits are prominent and transcortical sensory aphasias may occur. Hypersomnolence may result from local pressure on the reticular activating system of the rostral brain stem.

Cerebellar hemorrhage presents with headache, vertigo, vomiting and an inability to stand, and compression of the pons often causes peripheral facial weakness and horizontal gaze palsy. Gait and truncal ataxia, and ipsilateral limb ataxia, may be difficult to recognize in the acute phase. Hemorrhage into the pons almost always causes a reduced level of consciousness. Bilateral gaze paresis and quadriplegia are often present.

A uniform finding after intracerebral hemorrhage is that the prognosis is best predicted by the level of consciousness at presentation. This has led to widespread clinical application of numerical systems that grade severity, such as the widely used Glasgow Coma Scale. Not surprisingly, the volume of hematoma in supratentorial events is a predictor of survival and potential outcome. The amount of blood in the ventricular system is another factor of prognostic significance. The overall rate of mortality at 30 days is 35–50%.

The role of surgical evacuation in treatment is still a matter of dispute, and there are few randomized controlled trials to inform clinical practice. Operations tend to be carried out on less severely affected patients, and those with lobar and cerebellar hemorrhage fare better than those with bleeding centered on the basal ganglia. Small-scale trials of surgical treatment of putaminal hemorrhage have arrived at different conclusions.

Newer surgical techniques, mostly pioneered in Japan, include stereostatic drainage under CT guidance occasionally supplemented by aspiration after instillation of fibrinolytics. Here again, the younger and less severely affected patients appear to have the better outcomes. It is clear that large-scale randomized controlled trials need to be carried out to clarify the situation.

Vascular causes of dementia

The prevalence of vascular dementia is difficult to determine because the criteria for diagnosis are imprecise and vary widely. However, there is general agreement that vascular causes are most likely in patients aged 85 years or older. Recently, there has been a growing awareness that the most frequent vascular cause of dementia is white-matter ischemia and not multiple cerebral infarctions. Although Alzheimer's disease is undoubtedly the most common dementing process, it is not clear at present whether vascular disease or Lewy body dementia is the more frequent. Clinical dementia may be caused by a multi-infarct state, but the neuropathology is often complicated by the presence of more than one disease process. Histopathological studies have variously concluded that vascular factors may be involved in 10–40% of cases.

Clinical evidence of multiple infarcts may be adduced from mode of onset, fluctuating deficits, focal neurological symptoms and signs of emotional lability. With cerebral infarction, the site may be as important as the volume of brain lost. Multiple cortical infarcts caused by cardiogenic embolism may cause dementia; the most commonly seen clinical findings in these cases are aphasia, agnosia, apraxia and memory loss.

One infarct in a critical area may also cause dementia without multiple events[45]. Infarction of the angular gyrus in the inferior parietal lobule, for example, may cause dementia accompanied by Wernicke's aphasia, with or without right, left and finger agnosias, acalculia, agraphia and visuospatial abnormalities. Stroke in the ventromedial sector of the frontal lobes may have devastating effects on behavior by causing apathy and an inability to initiate either activity or conversation. Bilateral infarction of both caudate nuclei has similar effects.

Subcortical lacunar events causing dementia are characterized by psychomotor retardation and abulia combined with a shuffling gait (*marche à petit pas*), bilateral spasticity, dysphagia, dysarthria and emotional incontinence. Hypertension has been predictive of white-matter lesions on MRI in population surveys[46].

A rare genetic syndrome termed CADASIL (cerebral autosomal-dominant arteriopathy with subcortical infarcts and leukoencephalopathy) has recently been described in a number of European families with reported linkage to chromosome 19. Recurrent ischemic symptoms start at a relatively young age, and progress to pseudobulbar palsy and subcortical dementia, with death tending to occur within 10 years of presentation. MRI reveals a marked increase in signal intensity from subcortical white matter with multiple small deep infarcts, but sparing of the cerebral cortex.

The advent of modalities such as CT and especially MRI has drawn attention to the frequent occurrence of white-matter lesions in elderly patients. Periventricular low attenuation on CT, also referred to as leukoariosis, is common with advancing age, and probably represents demyelination and gliosis as a consequence of arteriosclerosis of the long penetrating end arterioles. The cerebral cortex presumably becomes disconnected as a consequence.

In a recent report by Langstreth and colleagues of a large population-based MRI study of cardiovascular health in elderly subjects[47], high-grade white-matter lesions were more often found in patients who presented with gait problems and cognitive decline. These results support the original concept of Binswanger's disease as being caused by chronic ischemia of the end arteries of the medulla.

The Cardiovascular Health Study has also shed light on the vexed question of the significance of so-called unidentified bright objects (UBOs). Punctate bilateral UBOs appear to correspond to dilated perivascular spaces around spirally elongated penetrating arteries. Lacunar infarcts in the basal ganglia, internal capsule, pons, thalamus and centrum ovale were also frequent findings.

Another finding of this study was that white-matter disease was more likely to be seen in patients with hypertension and vascular risk factors such as cigarette-smoking. Surprisingly, diabetes mellitus did not appear to be predictive of lesions. Follow-up studies in this cohort are likely to resolve many of the questions regarding the clinical significance of white-matter lesions seen on MRI.

Primary prevention

Hypertension

Arterial pressure is by far the best predictor of stroke and is implicated in the great majority of vascular events. There is incontrovertible evidence from large-scale randomized controlled trials that treatment of even mild-to-moderate hypertension is effective.

Collins and colleagues, in their meta-analysis of treatment trials of mild-to-moderate hypertension[48,49], found evidence of a reduction in incidence of fatal and non-fatal stroke that was proportional to the blood pressure-lowering achieved. The reduction in incidence was striking: almost all of the expected excess risk of a high blood pressure in causing stroke was prevented by effective anti-hypertensive treatment. Failures of prevention were related to failure of treatment to normalize blood pressure. There is also evidence that control of systolic hypertension in the elderly is effective in preventing stroke.

Smoking increases the risk of stroke substantially[50]; a recent meta-analysis has calculated that the population attributable risk for stroke is around 12%. Age, female gender and number of cigarettes smoked all appear to be relevant.

Diabetes may also increase the risk of stroke, although some conclude that its independent effect is in fact modest when hypertension, smoking and obesity are also taken into account[51]. In Finland, diabetic subjects appear to be at high risk of death from stroke[52]. Obesity is predictive of stroke and abdominal obesity, as determined by waist–hip ratio, may be particularly detrimental. Plasma fibrinogen, as in coronary heart disease, also appears to be a risk factor.

The relationship of stroke to serum cholesterol is generally much less convincing, although a clear inverse relationship between intracerebral hemorrhage and serum cholesterol has been consistently observed in Japanese populations. Increased cholesterol levels might be expected to increase atherothrombotic stroke by affecting internal carotid and large cerebral artery atherosclerosis, but clinical definition of this type of stroke is not always reliable.

At present, there is no convincing evidence that aspirin as primary prevention is beneficial, and there is indeed slight evidence from the British Doctors Trial that aspirin may predispose to more severe events[53]. The evidence regarding low-dose oral contraceptive use is inconclusive at present, although a definite increased risk has been recorded for the higher-dose preparations used in the past, especially in women aged >35 years who are smokers. A large-scale randomized controlled trial of hormone replacement therapy (HRT) is underway in the USA and should provide further information on stroke. The available data at present as regards risks or benefits are limited.

In conclusion, the cornerstone of any stratagem to prevent stroke is more effective treatment of arterial hypertension.

References

1. Malmgren R, Warlow C, Sandercock P, Slattery P. Geographical and secular trends in stroke incidence. *Lancet* 1987;ii:1196–1200

2. Bonita R, Stewart A, Beaglehole R. International trends in stroke mortalities: 1970–1985. *Stroke* 1990;21:989–92

3. Bonita R. Epidemiological studies and the prevention of stroke. *Cerebrovasc Dis* 1994;4 (Suppl 1):2–10

4. Eisenblätter D, Heinemann L, Classen E. Community-based stroke incidence trends from the 1970s through the 1980s in East Germany. *Stroke* 1995;26:919–23

5. Brown RD, Whisnant JP, Sicks JD, O'Fallon WM, Wiebers DO. Stroke incidence, prevalence and survival. *Stroke* 1996;27:373–80

6. Bamford J, Sandercock P, Dennis M, Burn J, Warlow C. Classification and national history of clinically identifiable subtypes of cerebral infarction. *Lancet* 1991;337:1521–6

7. Fisher CM. Lacunar infarcts – A review. *Cerebrovasc Dis* 1991;1:311–20

8. Kunitz SC, Gross CR, Heyman A, *et al.* The Pilot Stroke Data Bank: Definition, design, data. *Stroke* 1984;15:740–6

9. National Institute of Neurological Diseases and Stroke. Classification of cerebrovascular diseases. III. *Stroke* 1990;21:637–76

10. Ringelstein EB. Skepticism toward carotid ultrasonography: A virtue, an attitude or fanaticism. *Stroke* 1995;26:1743–6

11. Alexandrov AV, Bladin CF, Maggisano R, Norris JW. Measuring carotid stenosis: Time for a reappraisal. *Stroke* 1993;24:1292–6

12. Wilterdink JL, Feldmann F, Easton D, Ward R. Performance of carotid ultrasound in evaluating candidates for carotid endarterectomy is optimized by an approach based on clinical outcome rather than accuracy. *Stroke* 1996; 27:1094–8

13. European Carotid Surgery Trialists Collaborative Group. MRC European Carotid Surgery Trial: Interim results for symptomatic patients with severe (70–99%) or with mild (0–29%) carotid stenosis. *Lancet* 1991;337:1235–43

14. North American Symptomatic Carotid End-arterectomy Trial Collaborators. Beneficial effect of carotid endarterectomy in symptomatic patients with high-grade carotid stenosis. *N Engl J Med* 1991; 325:445–53

15. Mayberg MR, Wilson SE, Yatsu F, *et al*. Carotid endarterectomy and prevention of cerebral ischemia in symptomatic carotid stenosis: Veterans Affairs Cooperative Studies Program 309 Trialist Group. *JAMA* 1991;266:3289–44

16. Asymptomatic Carotid Atherosclerosis Study Group. Carotid endarterectomy for patients with asymptomatic internal carotid artery stenosis. *JAMA* 1995;273:1421–8

17. Paddock-Eliasziw LM, Eliasziw M, Barr HWK, *et al*. Long-term prognosis and the effect of carotid endarterectomy in patients with ipsilateral ischaemic events. *Neurology* 1996;47: 1158–62

18. Antiplatelet Trialists' Collaboration. Collaborative overview of randomised trials of antiplatelet therapy. I: Prevention of death, myocardial therapy in various categories of patients. *Br Med J* 1994;308:81–106

19. CAPRIE Steering Committee. A randomised, blinded, trial of clopidogrel versus aspirin in patients at risk of ischaemic events (CAPRIE). *Lancet* 1996;348:1329–39

20. Hart RG, Harrison MJG. Aspirin wars. The optimal dose of aspirin to prevent stroke. *Stroke* 1996;27:585–7

21. Barnett HJM, Kaste M, Meldrum H, Eliasziw M. Aspirin dose in stroke prevention. Beautiful hypothesis slain by ugly facts. *Stroke* 1996;27: 588–92

22. Chen J, Simon R. Ischaemic tolerance in the brain. *Neurology* 1997;48:306–11

23. Cerebral Embolism Task Force. Cardiogenic brain embolism: Second report of the Cerebral Embolism Task Force. *Arch Neurol* 1989;46: 727–41

24. Bogousslavsky J, Cachin C, Regli F, *et al*. Cardiac sources of embolism and cerebral infarction: Clinical consequences and vascular concomitants. *Neurology* 1991;41:855–9

25. Loh E, Sutton M St J, Wun C-CC, *et al*. Ventricular dysfunction and the risk of stroke after myocardial infarction. *N Engl J Med* 1997; 336:251–7

26. Sandercock PAG, Warlow CP, Jones LN, Starkey IR. Predisposing factors for cerebral infarction: The Oxfordshire Community Stroke Project. *Br Med J* 1989;298:75–80

27. Turpie AGG, Gent M, Laupacis A, *et al*. A comparison of aspirin with placebo in patients treated with warfarin after heart valve replacement. *N Engl J Med* 1993;19:524–9

28. Lechat P, Mas JL, Lascault G, *et al*. Prevalence of patent foramen ovale in patients with stroke. *N Engl J Med* 1988;318:1148–52

29. Jauss M, Kaps M, Keberle M, Haberbosch W, Dorndorf W. A comparison of transesophageal echocardiography and transcranial Doppler sonography with contrast medium for detection of patent foramen ovale. *Stroke* 1994;25:1265–7

30. The French Study of Aortic Plaques in Stroke Groups. Atherosclerotic disease of the aortic arch as a risk factor for recurrent ischemic stroke. *N Engl J Med* 1996;334:1216–21

31. The Boston Area Anticoagulation Trial for Atrial Fibrillation Investigators. The effect of low-dose warfarin on the risk of stroke in patients with non-rheumatic atrial fibrillation. *N Engl J Med* 1990;323:1505–11

32. Connolly SJ, Laupacis A, Gent M, Roberts RS, Cairns JA, Joyner C. Canadian Atrial Fibrillation Anticoagulation (CAFA) Study. *J Am Coll Cardiol* 1991;18:349–55

33. Ezekowitz MD, Bridgers SL, James KE, *et al.* Warfarin in the prevention of stroke associated with nonrheumatic atrial fibrillation. *N Engl J Med* 1992;327:1406–12 (Erratum *N Engl J Med* 1993; 328:148)

34. Peterson P, Godtfredson J, Anderson B, Boysen G, Anderson ED. Placebo-controlled, randomised trial of warfarin and aspirin for prevention of thromboembolic complications in chronic atrial fibrillation: The Copenhagen AFASAK Study. *Lancet* 1989;i:175–9

35. McBride R. Stroke Prevention in Atrial Fibrillation Study: Final results. *Circulation* 1991;84:527–39

36. EAFT (European Atrial Fibrillation Trial) Study Group. Secondary prevention in non-rheumatic atrial fibrillation after transient ischaemic attack in minor stroke. *Lancet* 1993;342:1255–62

37. European and Atrial Fibrillation Trial Study Groups. Optimal anticoagulant therapy in patients with nonrheumatic atrial fibrillation and recent cerebral ischemia. *N Engl J Med* 1995;333:5–10

38. Vaitkus PT, Barnathan ES. Embolic potential, prevention and management of mural thrombus complicating anterior myocardial infarction: A meta-analysis. *J Am Coll Cardiol* 1993;22:1004–9

39. Jorgensen HS, Nakayama H, Raaschou HO, Larsen K, Hubbe P, Olsen TS. The effect of a stroke unit: Reductions in mortality, discharge rate to nursing home, length of hospital stay and cost. A community-based study. *Stroke* 1995;26:1178–82

40. Smith DS, Goldenberg E, Ashburn A, *et al.* Remedial therapy after stroke: A randomised controlled trial. *BMJ* 1981;282:517–20

41. Strand T, Apslund K, Eriksson S, Hagg E, Lithner F, Wester PO. A non-intensive stroke unit reduces functional disability and the need for long-term hospitalization. *Stroke* 1985;16:29–34

42. Ween JE, Alexander MP, D'Esposito M, Roberts M. Factors predictive of stroke outcome in a rehabilitation setting. *Neurology* 1996;47:388–92

43. Vinters HV. Cerebral amyloid angiopathy. A critical review. *Stroke* 1987;18:311–21

44. Furlan AJ, Kanoti G. When is thrombolysis justified in patients with acute ischaemic stroke? *Stroke* 1997;28:214–8

45. Censori B, Manara O, Agostinis C, *et al.* Dementia after first stroke. Stroke 1996;27:1205–10

46. Liao D, Couper L, Cai J, *et al.* Presence and severity of cerebral white matter lesions and hypertension, its treatment, and its control. The ARIC Study. *Stroke* 1996;27:2262–70

47. Longstreth WT, Manolio TA, Arnold A, *et al.*, for the Cardiovascular Health Study Collaborative Research Group. Clinical correlates of white matter findings on cranial magnetic resonance imaging of 3,301 elderly people: The Cardiovascular Health Study. *Stroke* 1996;27:1274–82

48. Collins R, Peto R, MacMahon S, et al. Blood pressure, stroke and coronary heart disease. Part I. Prolonged differences in blood pressure: Prospective observational studies corrected for the regression dilution bias. Lancet 1990; 335:765–74

49. Collins R, Peto R, MacMahon S, et al. Blood pressure, stroke and coronary heart disease. Part II. Overview of randomised drug trials in their epidemiological context. Lancet 1990; 335:827–38

50. Wolf PA, D'Agostino RB, Kannel WB, Bonita R, Belanger AJ. Cigarette smoking as a risk factor for stroke: The Framingham Study. JAMA 1988; 259:1025–9

51. Welin L, Svärdsudd K, Wilhelmson L, Larsson B, Tibblin G. Analysis of risk factors for stroke in a cohort of men born in 1913. N Engl J Med 1987;317:521–6

52. Tuomilehto J, Rastenyte MD, Jousilahti P, Sarti C, Vartiainen E. Diabetes mellitus as a risk factor for death from stroke. Stroke 1996;27: 210–5

53. Peto R, Gray R, Collins R, et al. Randomised trial of prophylactic aspirin in British male doctors. Br Med J 1988;296:313–6

Further reading

Amar K, Wilcock G. Vascular dementia. *Br Med J* 1996;312:227–31

Bogousslavsky J, Caplan L, eds. *Stroke Syndromes.* Cambridge: Cambridge University Press, 1995

Bronner LL, Kanter DS, Manson JE. Primary prevention of stroke. *N Engl J Med* 1995;335:1392–1400

Brust JCM. Vascular dementia is overdiagnosed. *Arch Neurol* 1988;45:799-801

Jellinger K, Danielczyk W, Fischer P, Gabriel E. Clinicopathological analysis of dementia described in the elderly. *J Neurol Sci* 1990;95:239–58

Kase CS, Caplan LS, eds. *Intracerebral Haemorrhage.* Boston, London: Butterworth–Heinemann, 1994

Langhorne P, for Stroke Unit Triallists' Collaboration. Collaborative systematic review of the randomised trials of organised inpatient (stroke unit) care after stroke. *Br Med J* 1997;314:1151–9
O'Brien MD. Vascular dementia is underdiagnosed. *Arch Neurol* 1988;45:797–8

Stroke octet (series of papers)

Bamford J. Clinical examination in diagnosis and subclassification of stroke. *Lancet* 1992;339: 400–5

Bonita R. Epidemiology of stroke. *Lancet* 1992;339:342–4

Caplan LR. Intracerebral haemorrhage. *Lancet* 1992;339:656–8

Donnan GA. Investigation of patients with stroke and transient ischaemic attacks. *Lancet* 1992;339:473–7

van Gijn J. Subarachnoid haemorrhage. *Lancet* 1992;339:653–5

Hart RG. Cardiogenic embolism to the brain. *Lancet* 1992;339:489–594

Landi G. Clinical diagnosis of transient ischaemic attacks. *Lancet* 1992;339:402–5

Marmot MG, Poulter NR. Primary prevention of stroke. *Lancet* 1992;339:344–7

Oppenheimer S, Hachinski V. Complications of acute stroke. *Lancet* 1992;339:721–4

Pulsinelli W. Pathophysiology of acute ischaemic stroke. *Lancet* 1992;339:533–6

Sandercock P, Willems H. Medical treatment of acute ischaemic stroke. *Lancet* 1992;339:537–9

Section 2   Stroke Illustrated

List of illustrations

Classification of stroke (1)

Oxford

    Anterior circulation
        Total (TACI)
        Partial (PACI)

    Posterior circulation (POCI)

    Lacunar (LACI)

Stroke Data Bank

    Large artery atherosclerosis

    Lacunar

    Cardioembolic

    Tandem arterial lesions

    Unknown etiology

    Other

Figure 1 Two schemes for the classification of ischemic strokes

Classification of stroke (2)

National Institute of Neurological Diseases and Stroke

    Clinical

        Atherothrombotic
        Cardioembolic
        Lacunar

    Arterial territory

        Internal carotid
        Middle cerebral
        Anterior cerebral
        Vertebral
        Basilar
        Posterior cerebral

    Mechanism

        Thrombotic
        Embolic
        Hemodynamic

Figure 2 Another scheme for the classification of ischemic strokes

Figure 50
CT (same patient as in Figure 48) after 48 h shows extensive hemorrhagic transformation

Figure 51
Transesophageal echocardiogram showing left atrial thrombus and 'spontaneous contrast'

Figure 52
Transesophageal echocardiogram showing left atrial 'spontaneous contrast' or 'smoke'

Figure 53
Transthoracic echocardiogram showing a dilated left ventricle

Figure 54
Transthoracic echocardiogram showing thrombus in the left ventricle

Figure 55
Transthoracic echocardiogram with Doppler signature showing markedly increased aortic systolic flow velocity

Figure 56
Transesophageal echocardiogram showing vegetation on the mitral valve

Figure 57
CDI showing shunting of blood through patent foramen ovale

Figure 58
Transesophageal echocardiogram showing a myxoma in the left atrium

Figure 59
Transesophageal echocardiogram showing an aneurysm of the interatrial septum

Figure 60
Transesophageal echocardiogram showing Chiari network in the left atrium

Figure 61
CT showing small area of increased attenuation in the right basal ganglia

Figure 62
CT showing lacunar infarct in the right basis pontis

Figure 63
CT showing lacunar infarct of right lateral thalamus

Figure 64
CT showing tiny deep infarct in the left internal capsule

Figure 65
CT showing bilateral lacunar strokes

Figure 66
CT showing small deep-lying hemorrhage which may present identically to a lacunar infarct

Figure 67
T_2-weighted MRI showing lacunar infarcts of anterior poles of the right thalamus

Figure 68
CT showing striatocapsular infarct involving caudate nucleus and internal capsule

Figure 69
ECG in severe hypertension showing left ventricular hypertrophy

Figure 70
CT showing periventricular attenuation due to diffuse white-matter ischemia

Figure 71
CT (same patient as in Figure 70) showing reduced attenuation around anterior horns of lateral ventricles

Figure 72
T_2-weighted MRI showing extensive periventricular white-matter ischemia

Figure 73
3-D surface reconstruction of spiral CT angiogram showing normal circle of Willis

Figure 74
MRI angiogram showing a normal circle of Willis

Figure 75
CT showing blood in the subarachnoid space

Figure 76
CT (same patient as in Figure 75) shows hematoma in the ventromedial frontal lobe

Figure 77
MRI angiogram (same patient as in Figure 75) showing aneurysm of the anterior communicating artery

Classification of stroke (1)

Oxford

    Anterior circulation
        Total (TACI)
        Partial (PACI)

    Posterior circulation (POCI)

    Lacunar (LACI)

Stroke Data Bank

    Large artery atherosclerosis

    Lacunar

    Cardioembolic

    Tandem arterial lesions

    Unknown etiology

    Other

Figure 1 Two schemes for the classification of ischemic strokes

Classification of stroke (2)

National Institute of Neurological Diseases and Stroke

    Clinical
        Atherothrombotic
        Cardioembolic
        Lacunar

    Arterial territory
        Internal carotid
        Middle cerebral
        Anterior cerebral
        Vertebral
        Basilar
        Posterior cerebral

    Mechanism
        Thrombotic
        Embolic
        Hemodynamic

Figure 2 Another scheme for the classification of ischemic strokes

Causes of acute ischemic stroke and transient ischemic attacks (1)

Atherothrombosis

Disease of small medullary arteries

> Hypertension
>
> Diabetes mellitus
>
> CADASIL syndrome: Familial syndrome with autosomal dominant inheritance leading to early subcortical stroke and vascular dementia

Necrotizing arteritis (including Takayasu's disease)

Arterial dissection (trauma, but may be familial)

Cardiac embolism due to
> Acute myocardial infarction (especially anterior)
> LV aneurysm, dyskinetic segment
> Poor function
> Atrial dilatation / fibrillation
> Infective endocarditis
> Non-infective endocarditis
> Atrial myxoma

Artery-to-artery embolism due to
> Atherosclerosis of aorta or of large arteries, including arterial dissection

Paradoxical embolism
> Thrombophilias, including factor V Leiden

Vasospasm
> Migraine
> Drug-induced

Figure 3 Vascular causes of ischemic stroke

Causes of acute ischemic stroke and transient ischemic attacks (2)

Systemic infections, especially pneumonia

Systemic lupus erythematosus

Thrombocytosis and myeloproliferative diseases

Thrombophilias
(much more likely to develop cerebral venous thrombosis)
> Factor V Leiden
> Deficiency of protein C or S

Figure 4 Blood disorders predisposing to ischemic stroke

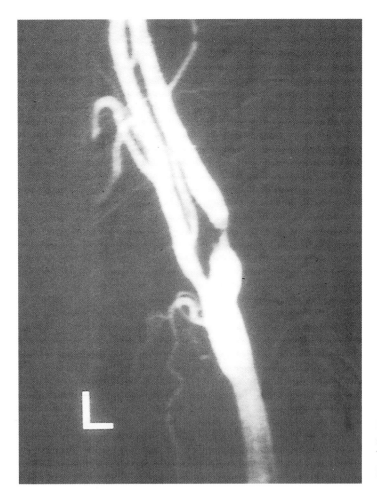

Figure 5 Angiogram showing a severe stenosis in the left internal carotid artery. The patient presented with a transient right hemiparesis

Figure 6 Funduscopy showing a central retinal artery occlusion, a condition that is usually due to atheroembolism. The evidence for an artery-to-artery embolism in this retina is the refractile so-called Hollenhorst plaque lodged at a point of arterial bifurcation in the nasal retina (arrowed). Amaurosis fugax is commonly the result of embolism from an internal carotid artery stenosis

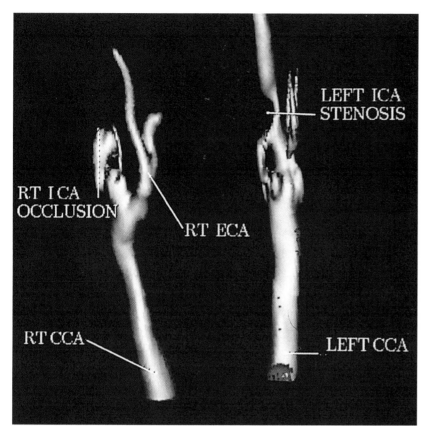

Figure 7 Three-dimensional (3-D) surface reconstruction of spiral CT angiogram in a patient with hemiplegia due to an infarct in the territory of the right middle cerebral artery. There is occlusion of the right internal carotid artery and a tight stenosis of the left internal carotid artery

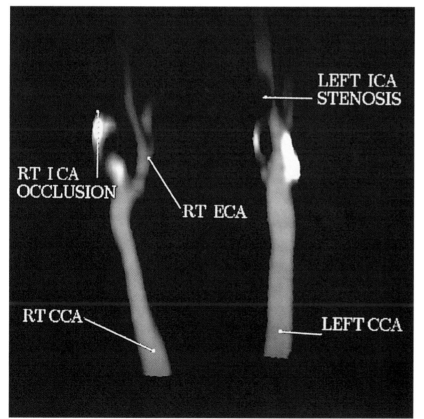

Figure 8 Maximum-intensity projection of the same scan as in Figure 7 clearly shows both lesions as well as areas of vascular calcification

Figure 9 Coronal section of cerebral cortex showing softening due to infarction in the territory of the left middle cerebral artery. The putamen is clearly involved. The corresponding clinical syndrome is often referred to as a total anterior circulation infarct (TACI), and is associated with a poor prognosis for survival and functional outcome

Figure 10 This internal carotid artery is occluded with thrombus superimposed on an atherosclerotic plaque. Approximately 30% of infarcts in the middle cerebral artery territory are caused by extracranial arterial disease. Depending on the adequacy of collateral flow and especially on the size of the posterior communicating artery, the extent of infarction after carotid occlusion varies considerably

Figure 11 Color Doppler imaging (CDI) of a normal carotid bifurcation. The common carotid artery (on the right) is clearly seen dividing into the internal (lower left) and external (upper left) carotid arteries. Normal flow velocity appears blue

Figure 12 CDI of a stenosis at the origin of the internal carotid artery. The common carotid artery (on the right) has a normal velocity of flow indicated by red. Increased velocities of flow through and distal to the stenosis are visualized as yellow and green

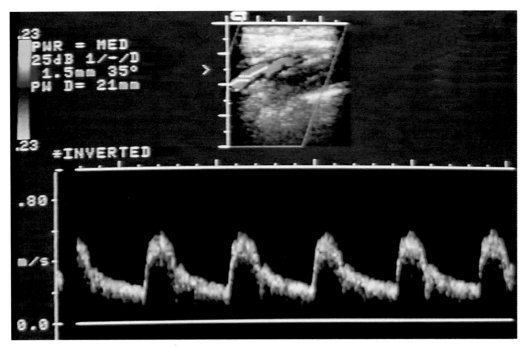

Figure 13 CDI of an internal carotid artery with normal flow velocity (shown by red). The Doppler signatures in the artery through several cardiac cycles are displayed below. The pulsed Doppler frequency spectrum shows a narrow range of frequencies with rounded peaks during systole and an average velocity 0.6 m/s (normal < 1.0)

Figure 14 CDI showing Doppler signatures of a severely stenosed internal carotid artery. There is a marked increase in peak velocity to > 6 m/s (normal < 1.0) and a sharp peak. Flow disturbance is also indicated by the much wider range of velocities reflected by the broadening of the spectrum compared with normal

Figure 15 CT showing border-zone or 'watershed' cortical infarcts in a patient with occlusion of the right internal carotid artery. The border zones between the territories of the middle and anterior cerebral arteries, and middle and posterior cerebral arteries, respectively, are vulnerable when carotid pressure is greatly reduced. As there is considerable variation among individuals in respective arterial territories, border-zone infarcts are not always as easy to recognize

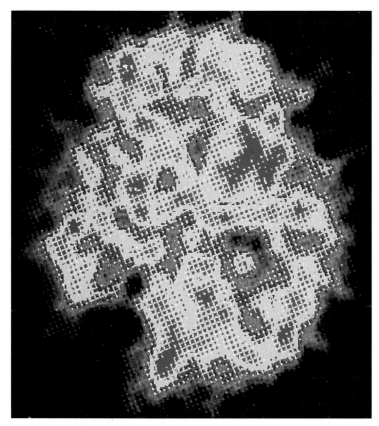

Figure 16 Technetium 99m-hexamethyl-propylene amine oxide (HMPAO) and single-photon emission tomography (SPECT) (same patient as in Figure 15) showing the area of reduced perfusion associated with the more posterior infarct. More anteriorly, a smaller area of reduced perfusion is just discernible

Figure 17 Focal seizures causing hemi-sensory symptoms may be mistaken for transient ischemic attacks (TIAs). This parietal meningioma, shown here on T_2-weighted MRI, resulted in left-sided symptoms which were misdiagnosed as TIAs

Figure 18 CT showing infarction in the territory of the central branch of the left middle cerebral artery which presented as mild weakness and numbness of the right arm. The infarct was probably caused by artery-to-artery embolism from a proximal internal carotid stenosis

Figure 19 Early changes of infarction are difficult to detect on CT. In this 34-year-old patient, increased attenuation can be seen in the right middle cerebral artery territory due to increased water content of ischemic tissue. There is loss of definition of the corresponding lentiform nucleus (normal nucleus is arrowed)

Figure 20 On CT, another useful sign of infarction can be seen here in the territory of the middle cerebral artery – loss of the ribbon deep in the Sylvian fissure (normal ribbon is arrowed)

Figure 21 CT showing middle cerebral artery occlusion. There is increased attenuation in the stem of the artery, referred to as the 'string sign'

Figure 22 Angiography (same patient as in Figure 21) shows thrombus (arrowed) causing partial occlusion of the proximal middle cerebral artery

Figure 23 CT showing a 'dense' and probably calcified middle cerebral artery which can be seen particularly clearly against the old infarct in the corresponding territory

Figure 24 CT showing an infarct that is both deep and superficial in the left middle cerebral artery territory, and which has undergone hemorrhagic transformation in the region of the caudate nucleus. The scan was prompted by clinical deterioration 3 days after the onset of hemiplegia. Larger infarcts are more susceptible to hemorrhage

Figure 25 Transcranial CDI signature demonstrating a normal spectrum of velocities in the middle cerebral artery

Figure 26 Transcranial CDI signature of a middle cerebral artery shows a highly abnormal pattern with much increased velocities as a result of partial occlusion

Figure 27 Carotid angiogram of an 18-year-old girl who had recurrent cerebral ischemic events showing neovascularization at the base of the brain and extending posteriorly. The 'puff of smoke' appearance is diagnostic of moyamoya syndrome

Figure 28 Transesophageal echocardiography showing an aortic dissection extending to the distal arch. The intimal flap is clearly seen (arrowed), and there is thrombus in the false lumen to the left and above. Aortic dissection is an uncommon cause of cerebral infarction and an occasional cause of spinal cord infarction

Figure 29 T$_1$-weighted MRI showing infarction of the cerebellum and lateral medulla in the territory supplied by the posterior inferior cerebellar artery and causing Wallenberg's syndrome. Occlusion in such cases is usually proximal in the vertebral artery and may be due to either atherosclerosis or cardioembolism. Dissection of the vertebral artery in the neck, sometimes caused by trauma, is a relatively rare but well-recognized cause

Figure 30 T$_2$-weighted MRI showing infarction confined to the lateral medulla, the result of vertebral artery occlusion

Figure 31 T$_2$-weighted MRI showing infarction of the cerebellum in the territory of the anterior inferior cerebellar artery. This sometimes leads to a clinical syndrome which is characterized by ipsilateral incoordination, tinnitus, dysarthria, facial weakness, hearing loss, loss of sensation in the trigeminal area, Horner's syndrome and contralateral loss of spinothalamic sensation

Figure 32 T$_2$-weighted MRI showing bilateral infarction of the cerebellum due to cardioembolism. Infarction that is confined to the superior cerebellar artery is usually a result of embolism

Figure 33 T$_1$-weighted MRI of a 52-year-old hypertensive cigarette smoker who has developed brain-stem infarction due to basilar artery occlusion. There is extensive infarction of the pons and right superior cerebellum. By this stage of disease, the patient showed quadriplegia and skew deviation of the eyes

Figure 34 T$_1$-weighted MRI (same patient as in Figure 33) at a lower level shows widespread patchy cerebellar infarction

Figure 35 CTs showing infarction due to embolic occlusion of the basilar artery which is particularly marked in both cerebellar hemispheres as well as in the lower part of the left temporal lobe (upper) and in the occipital cortex (lower)

Figure 36 T$_2$-weighted MRI of a hypertensive patient who developed a small midbrain infarct. The clinical features included a right oculomotor palsy and contralateral incoordination (Claude's syndrome)

Figure 37 CT showing atherothrombotic occlusion of the posterior cerebral artery which has resulted in an infarction of the occipital cortex extending to the temporal lobe. Clinical features included agitation, persistent amnesia and a Wernicke's aphasia of transcortical type

Figure 38 CT showing infarction of the left occipital cortex with resultant hemianopia in a 58-year-old patient with thrombophlebitis migrans subsequently shown to be associated with metastatic carcinoma of the pancreas

Figure 39 CT (same patient as in Figure 38) showing the later development of an infarction of the contralateral occipital cortex which left the patient with only central vision. It is likely that a coagulopathy was responsible, although cardioembolism was also considered

Figure 40 CT of a 33-year-old patient who presented with sudden-onset severe motor hemiplegia. The infarction is predominantly striatocapsular, characteristic of occlusion of the proximal middle cerebral artery and usually the result of embolism. Within the infarct, there is a small area of hemorrhagic transformation

Figure 41 CT (same patient as in Figure 40) taken on the following day shows that the hemorrhagic transformation has become more extensive, presumably due to reperfusion

Figure 42 T$_2$-weighted MRI (same patient as in Figure 40) taken 4 days after onset shows hemorrhage surrounded by edema or infarction. There is also evidence of ischemia in the peripheral territories of the middle cerebral artery

Figure 43 MRI angiography (same patient as in Figure 40) taken at the same stage of disease shows that middle cerebral artery patency has been restored

Figure 44 CDI shows normal flow in the external carotid artery (orange) whereas the internal carotid artery (below and to the left) is occluded by thrombus which, in this case, was due to embolism from an acute anterior myocardial infarction

Figure 45 Angiogram of the left carotid artery showing an absence of flow in the lower division of the middle cerebral artery due to cardiogenic embolism. Strokes of this type usually result in Wernicke's aphasia and are most often due to cardiogenic or artery-to-artery embolism

Figure 46 Transesophageal echocardiography of an 80-year-old patient who had atrial flutter / fibrillation and multiple cerebral infarcts on CT. A mobile thrombus (arrowed) can be seen in the left atrial appendage

Figure 47 CT (same patient as in Figure 46) showing cerebral cortical infarcts. The infarct in the occipital lobe is old whereas that in the superficial middle cerebral territory is relatively recent. Both were caused by embolism

Figure 48 Transesophageal echocardiography of a 50-year-old patient 3 weeks after Q-wave anterior myocardial infarction reveals a mass of thrombus (arrowed) in an aneurysmal dilatation at the apex of the left ventricle

Figure 49 CT (same patient as in Figure 48) showing early changes of infarction in the right middle cerebral artery territory after sudden onset of left hemiplegia, hemisensory loss and hemianopia

Figure 50 CT (same patient as in Figure 48) after clinical deterioration 48 h later shows extensive hemorrhagic transformation. Infarcts resulting from embolism are prone to such transformation

Figure 51 Transesophageal echocardiography of a 57-year-old patient with atrial fibrillation who developed a severe posterior circulation stroke due to cardiogenic embolism. There is thrombus (arrowed) in the left atrium and adjacent 'spontaneous contrast', an appearance which is probably the result of stagnant blood flow

Figure 52 Transesophageal echocardiography showing the appearance of 'spontaneous contrast' (arrowed) in the left atrium of a patient with atrial fibrillation and suspected embolic stroke

Figure 53 Transthoracic echocardiography in a patient with dilated cardiomyopathy shows a greatly enlarged left ventricle (arrowed) which was contracting very poorly. The risk of embolic stroke in this type of patient is high

Figure 54 Transthoracic echocardiography of a patient following anterior myocardial infarction demonstrates a thrombus (arrowed) in the left ventricle. Anterior myocardial infarction carries a much higher risk of embolism compared with inferior infarction

Figure 55 Transthoracic echocardiography with Doppler signature showing markedly increased aortic systolic flow, reaching nearly 6 m / s, due to severe aortic stenosis. Calcific aortic stenosis and mitral annulus calcification have been suspected to cause embolic stroke

Figure 56 Transesophageal echocardiography showing a vegetation (arrowed) on the posterior leaflet of the mitral valve. Vegetations due to infective endocarditis may cause embolic stroke

Figure 57 CDI showing shunting of blood from the right to left atrium via a patent foramen ovale (arrowed). The increased velocity of blood flow is indicated by yellow. Patients with shunts are at risk of paradoxical embolism. Another technique to demonstrate this type of shunt uses transcranial Doppler monitoring after intravenous injection of microbubbles

Figure 58 Transesophageal echocardiography showing a large left atrial myxoma (arrowed) in a patient who presented with transient cerebral ischemic attacks presumably due to emboli from the tumor

Figure 59 Transesophageal echocardiography showing an aneurysmal area in the interatrial septum (arrowed), seen bulging towards the right atrium, of a patient who presented with transient ischemic attacks. Abnormalities in this area may predispose to embolism

Figure 60 Transesophageal echocardiography showing a filamentous structure or Chiari network (arrowed) in the left atrium. Such an appearance has been suspected to predispose to embolism

Figure 61 CT showing a small area of increased attenuation in the right basal ganglia due to a small deeply lying infarct, resulting from occlusion of a single penetrating artery. The pathological term lacune is used to describe a slit-like space in deep-lying white matter caused by single penetrating artery occlusion, small hemorrhages or a dilated perivascular space

Figure 62 CT showing a lacunar infarct of the right basis pontis in a 41-year-old patient presenting with ataxic hemiparesis on the left side. The patient had severe hypertension

Figure 63 CT showing a lacunar infarct of the right lateral thalamus in a 51-year-old patient with severe hypertension who presented with pure sensory stroke. The infarct has probably resulted from an occlusion of a perforator from the thalamogeniculate artery originating from the posterior cerebral artery

Figure 64 CT showing a very small deep infarct in the left internal capsule in a 63-year-old patient with hypertension and a transient (<24h) pure motor weakness affecting the contralateral face, arm and leg. Many such lacunar infarcts are clinically silent, but a transient ischemic attack may occur in around 20% of patients

Figure 65 CT showing bilateral lacunar strokes in a 70-year-old patient with treatment-resistant hypertension and renal impairment due to hypertensive nephrosclerosis. The presenting features were a shuffling gait and pseudobulbar palsy

Figure 66 CT showing a small deep-lying hemorrhage which may present identically to lacunar infarction. In this case, the clinical presentation suggested a sensorimotor lacunar stroke. Both entities result from the occlusion and rupture, respectively, of perforating end arteries and are frequently due to hypertension

Figure 67 T$_2$-weighted MRI of a 60-year-old taxi driver, who had poorly controlled hypertension and previous right hemi-paresis due to pure motor stroke, shows lacunar infarcts affecting the anterior poles of the thalamus, especially on the right. The patient presented with sudden-onset anterograde amnesia

Figure 68 CT showing a striatocapsular infarct involving the caudate nucleus, and anterior limb and genu of the internal capsule. The patient was a 52-year-old Chinese restaurateur who was a cigarette smoker with hypertension. Such infarcts sometimes present clinically as lacunar events, but are due to occlusive disease within the main stem of the middle cerebral artery. The clinical findings were agitation, dysarthria, central facial weak-ness and transient mild arm weakness

Figure 69 ECG in severe hypertension showing left ventricular hypertrophy by limb and chest lead-voltage criteria. Repolarization changes in the lateral leads or ST depression are often described as a 'strain' pattern: the S wave in VI plus R wave in V5 > 35 mm; the R wave in I plus S wave in III > 25 mm; the R wave in aVL > II mm

Figure 70 CT showing diffuse white-matter ischemia, which causes periventricular low attenuation. However, MRI is a more sensitive technique for visualizing these abnormalities. Age is the main predictor of this CT appearance

Figure 71 CT (same patient as in Figure 70) showing the reduced attenuation around the anterior horns of the lateral ventricles

Figure 72 T$_2$-weighted MRI showing extensive periventricular white-matter ischemia in a 79-year-old patient who presented with a shuffling gait, abulia, bilateral pyramidal signs, primitive reflexes and mild memory loss. The scan appearances are consistent with Binswanger's disease or microvascular ischemic leuko-encephalopathy

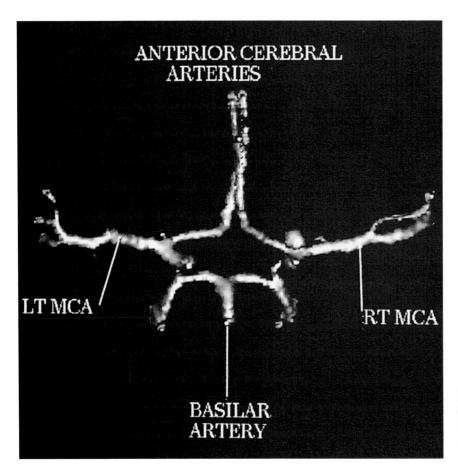

Figure 73 Three-dimensional surface reconstruction of a spiral CT shows a normal circle of Willis

Figure 74 MRI angiography does not use contrast and is able to produce surprisingly good views of the circle of Willis, as seen in this normal examination. The definition, however, is not as good as with contrast arteriography

Figure 75 CT showing blood in the subarachnoid space in a 68-year-old patient who presented with sudden-onset severe headache and vomiting, followed by agitation and amnesia. Negative findings on CT do not exclude subarachnoid hemorrhage

Figure 76 CT (same patient as in Figure 75) at a lower cut shows hematoma that extends forwards from the midline to the ventromedial frontal lobe. These appearances are characteristic of rupture of an aneurysm of the anterior communicating artery

Figure 77 MRI angiography (same patient as in Figure 75) showing a large 'berry' aneurysm of the anterior communicating artery. The circle of Willis is viewed from behind

Figure 78 Coronal section through the cerebral cortex shows recent cerebral hemorrhage centered on the basal ganglia in a patient with hypertension. The bleeding probably originated from a ruptured microaneurysm

Figure 79 CT showing a typical hemorrhage into the putamen in a 43-year-old patient with undiagnosed hypertension presenting with abrupt onset of hemiplegia, hemisensory loss, hemianopia, global aphasia and forced deviation of gaze to the left. Bleeding originated in the lateral lenticulostriate territory often called the artery of cerebral hemorrhage

Figure 80 CT showing a smaller hemorrhage in a 59-year-old patient with hypertension who presented with contralateral pure motor hemiparesis. In such cases, CT is essential for the diagnosis

Figure 81 CT appearance of the hemorrhage (upper left) is compared with T_1-weighted (upper right) and T_2-weighted (lower) MRIs taken in three planes (same patient as in Figure 80) during the acute stage. Note the increased signal intensity caused by edema around the hematoma in the T_1-weighted image

Figure 82 CT showing lobar intracerebral hemorrhage in the occipital cortex which presented as hemianopia, occipital headache and agitation in an 80-year-old patient. Bleeding at this age is often caused by amyloid angiopathy, which selectively affects small- and medium-sized arteries and veins of the cerebral cortex and pia mater

Figure 83 CT of intracerebral hemorrhage into the frontal lobe of an 82-year-old patient who presented with frontal headache, abulia, and weakness of the left arm and leg followed by seizures. On examination, there was a tendency towards rightward gaze. Amyloid angiopathy was suspected

Figure 84 CT of a hematoma in the left parietal lobe in a 90-year-old patient due to amyloid angiopathy. Hemorrhage of this type carries a relatively good short-term prognosis, but there is a high risk of recurrence. Note the apparent extension of the anterior horn of the left lateral ventricle due to previous hemorrhage into the frontal lobe

Figure 85 CT of a parieto-occipital lobar hemorrhage shows a layered appearance. Hemorrhage due to amyloid angiopathy often gives such an appearance, which may reflect a multicentric origin

Figure 86 CT showing hemorrhage into the right parietal lobe of an 81-year-old patient treated with warfarin as prophylaxis for cerebral embolism due to atrial fibrillation. Lobar hemorrhage may be caused by fibrinolytic or anticoagulant treatment

Figure 87 T$_2$-weighted MRI (same patient as in Figure 86) of the lobar hemorrhage in the subacute phase

Figure 88 Brain viewed from the base showing hemorrhage into the right lobe of the cerebellum

Figure 89 CT showing hemorrhage into the cerebellum, which may be caused by hypertension or amyloid angiopathy. The 62-year-old patient had poorly controlled hypertension and presented with collapse, inability to walk, occipital headache and vomiting. There was right-sided facial weakness of peripheral-type and gaze failure resulting from compression of the pons

Figure 90 Histology of the cerebral cortex showing a vessel stained to reveal amyloid in the vessel walls (Congo red & hematoxylin)

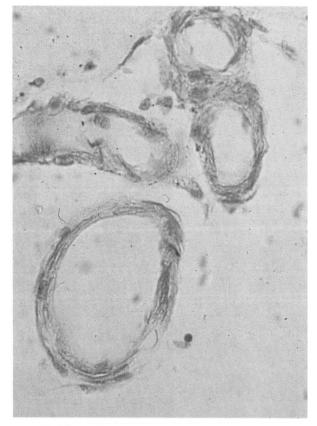

Figure 91 Histology of the leptomeninges showing vessels stained to reveal amyloid (Congo red & hematoxylin)

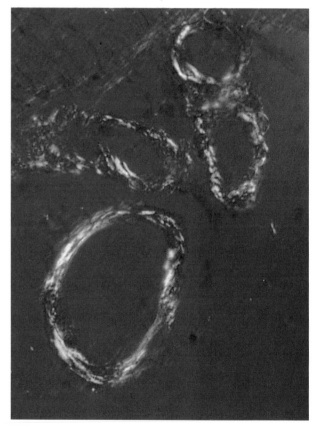

Figure 92 Histology of the leptomeninges showing vessels stained to reveal amyloid and viewed under polarized light to show the characteristic apple-green color (Congo red & hematoxylin)

Figure 93 CT showing an acute subdural hematoma causing appreciable midline shift in a 63-year-old patient who presented with aphasia and mild right hemiparesis. There was a background history of alcohol abuse and a minor head injury 4 days earlier

Figure 94 CT showing a less recent subdural hematoma which has become isodense with the brain tissue, although a hyperintense layer of more recent hemorrhage can still be seen adjacent to the cerebral cortex. Note the characteristic shape of the adjacent anterior horn of the lateral ventricle, which is often a clue to the presence of subdural blood on CT

Figure 95 CT after intravenous injection of contrast shows a left parieto-occipital arteriovenous malformation. Such lesions often cause lobar hematoma in younger patients. In this case, the malformation appears to be supplied by the left posterior cerebral artery

Figure 96 Contrast angiography (same patient as in Figure 95) of the vertebral artery confirms that the malformation is supplied by the left posterior cerebral artery. Lesions of this type also cause seizures

Figure 97 CT showing a left parietal hemorrhage in a 42-year-old patient with *Staphylococcus aureus* septicemia

Figure 98 CT (same patient as in Figure 97) at a higher cut shows a separate large frontoparietal hemorrhage. Bleeding as a result of septic embolism tends to originate from the junction between gray and white matter

Index

References to illustrations are shown in **bold**.